Contents

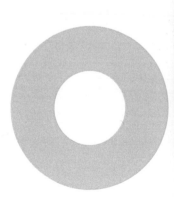

Self-Care and You
Starting Your Journey

A high quality life starts with a high quality you.
—Cheryl Richardson

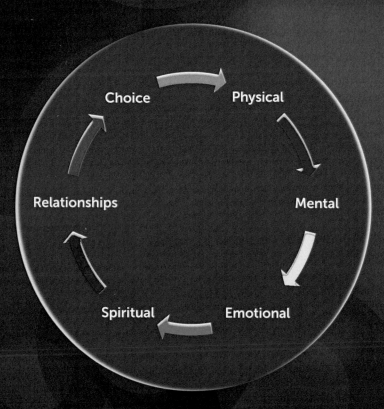

Choice
Physical
Mental
Emotional
Spiritual
Relationships

Six Self-Care Pathways

The practice of self-care is a lifelong journey. *Self-care* means choosing behaviors that balance the effects of emotional and physical stressors. These behaviors can include exercising, eating nutritious foods, getting enough sleep, practicing self-centering activities, abstaining from substance abuse, and pursuing creative outlets.

If you want to live a life of meaningful contribution to others, you may need to make changes in your own life first. Many caregivers fall into the trap of over-giving and wrongfully believing that self-care is selfish. Nothing could be further from the truth. The Code of Ethics for Nurses clearly supports this: "The nurse owes the same duty to self as to others, including the responsibility to preserve integrity and safety, to maintain competence, and to continue personal and professional growth" (ANA, 2001, p. 23). The reward for tending to your needs first is profound. You will find more passion, energy, and resilience to support making a difference in others' lives.

The practice of self-care means engaging in meaningful and nontoxic connections with others who support you, listening to your body when you feel something is awry, and knowing when you are headed toward exhaustion. Learning to *self-soothe,* or calm your physical and emotional distress, is also essential to self-care. While some routines will become a self-nurturing sanctuary, successful self-care journeys include dynamic change, adaptation, and flexibility.

Jeffrey Bland, a leader in nutritional medicine, has noted that at least 70% of all diseases are preventable or modifiable through lifestyle intervention (Bland, 2012). Bland points out that while we cannot control our genes, we can control the environment that allows wellness or disease to flourish. This field of study is defined as epigenetics. In other words, our everyday habits and stressors can control our "book of life."

Your Six Self-Care Pathways

Dossey and Keegan (2009) have identified the importance of self-care by utilizing six key pathways, or elements, of self-care: physical, mental, emotional, spiritual, relationship, and choice. As we delve into each pathway, it will become clear that they are interconnected. The natural interweaving, multi-directional flow of each pathway serves to boost or hinder other pathways; the diagram on the opposite page illustrates one level of these interactions.

A profound example of this relationship can be seen in a study focused specifically on the likelihood of an acute myocardial infarction (MI) in the immediate period after the death of someone close. Researchers found a staggering 21-fold increased risk of an MI in the first 24 hours of learning of the death of a significant other compared with other times (Mostofsky et al., 2012). The impact of emotional, spiritual, and mental well-being is undeniably connected with physiological dynamics in the body. Psychological stress, such as that caused by intense grief, can raise the heart rate and increase blood pressure and coagulation—factors that contribute to the risk of an MI. The bereaved are also more likely to neglect taking regular medications, as well as experience less sleep, a decreased appetite, and high cortisol levels, all of which can increase the probability of an MI.

Compassion Fatigue and Burnout

Health is not only to be well, but to use well every power we have. The martyr sacrifices themselves entirely in vain. Or rather not in vain: for they make the selfish more selfish, the lazy more lazy, the narrow narrower.

—Florence Nightingale

The visionary Florence Nightingale said it well. As nurses, our need to consistently give requires energy, resiliency, and mandatory refilling of our personal reservoirs. Soul-nurturing, life-affirming activities that reignite the spirit, cultivate compassion, and improve engagement are as important to the nursing profession as oxygen is to the lungs. The inherent desire to deeply care for others can put nurses at risk of compassion fatigue and burnout.

Figley (2002), a pioneer in the concept of compassion fatigue, has described compassion fatigue as a state experienced by individuals helping people in distress; it is an extreme state of tension and preoccupation with suffering. The helper, in contrast to the person(s) being helped, is traumatized or suffers due to the helper's own efforts to empathize and be compassionate. Often, this leads to poor self-care and extreme self-sacrifice. Figley believes that this combination can lead to compassion fatigue and symptoms similar to posttraumatic stress disorder (PTSD) (Gould, 2005).

Figley (2002) asserts that compassion fatigue is a construct of ten concepts:

- **Exposure to client** (direct care at high risk);
- **Empathic ability** (ability to sense pain);
- **Empathic concern** (motivation to respond);
- **Empathic response** (amount of effort to expend);
- **Residual compassion stress**;
- **Sense of achievement** (can buffer impact of compassion fatigue);
- **Disengagement** (ability to keep good boundaries);
- **Prolonged exposure**;
- **Traumatic recollection**; and
- **Degree of life disruption and other life demands**.

Sabo (2006) describes compassion fatigue as a severe malaise resulting from caring for patients that are experiencing varying aspects of pain (i.e., physical, emotional, social). Compassion fatigue is associated with the "cost of caring" and refers to the resultant strain and weariness that evolves over time (Showalter, 2010; Thomas & Wilson, 2004). Implicit in its nature is a preoccupation with the trauma experienced by patients (Figley, 2002). Compassion fatigue reduces the capacity of caregivers to empathize with patients due to prolonged exposure to suffering individuals (Meadors, Lamson, Swanson, White, & Sira, 2009).

Personal qualities that contribute to the risk of compassion fatigue include inadequate professional boundaries, unrealistic expectations, personal life events like divorce or bereavement, history of personal trauma, ineffective coping style, and untreated anxiety or depression (Yoder, 2010). Heavy workload, a lack of leadership, support, and autonomy, shift work (12 hours per day, 6 days per week), and experience with patients at end of life are also professional variables that contribute to the risk of compassion fatigue (Hooper, Craig, Janvin, Wetsel, & Reimels, 2010).

Burnout is the individual's defense response to prolonged interpersonal demand. Burnout results in withdrawal from the professional caregiver's role (Meadors et al., 2009), emotional and physical exhaustion for clinicians, and feelings of cynicism, detachment, and lack of personal accomplishment (Kearney, Weininger, Vachon, Harrison, & Mount, 2009). Symptoms for those suffering from burnout include irritability, impaired concentration, lethargy, illness, absence from work, substance abuse, and an increased likelihood of leaving their job (Absolon & Krueger, 2009).

> The inherent desire to deeply care for others can put nurses at risk of compassion fatigue and burnout, which can also affect patients and organizations.

Compassion fatigue and burnout are consequences for empathetic caregivers who do not make replenishment of self a priority within their professional role. The cost of compassion fatigue and burnout extends to nurse, patient, and organizational outcomes. Nurse outcomes include forgetfulness, losing things, anger, edginess, insomnia, depression, apathy, poor job morale and performance, increased sick calls, and leaving the profession (Absolon & Krueger, 2009). Specific physical manifestations of compassion fatigue include headaches, increased blood pressure, weight gain, diabetes, gastrointestinal conditions, and immune dysfunction (Aycock & Boyle, 2009). Compassion fatigue has also resulted in clinicians treating patients in an uncaring way (Aycock & Boyle, 2009). Each of these negative outcomes ends up resulting in an increase in the cost of care to mediate the negative outcomes on nurses and patients.

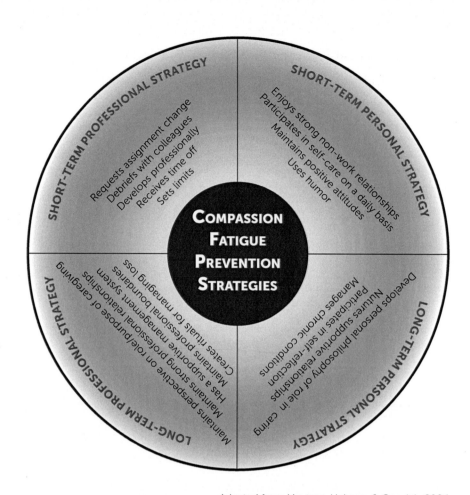

Adapted from Maytum, Heiman, & Garwick, 2004

Self-care has been shown to have a moderately-strong negative relationship with both compassion fatigue ($r = .60$, $p < .001$) and burnout ($r = .60$, $p < .001$) in a recent study of 65 staff nurses (Johnson, 2012). This study suggests that self-care is the antidote to compassion fatigue.

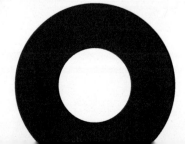

Compassion fatigue prevention strategies, both professional and personal, and long-term and short-term, are illustrated in the diagram above. Allotting time for yourself reduces your risk for compassion fatigue because self-care practices create more resilience, more flexibility, and more empathy for others.

About This Book

This book applies an integrated, holistic approach to the practice of self-care. The following sections on the six pathways are filled with tips, suggestions, guidelines, and examples to supplement the main text. As you read the book, consider using the Self-Care Assessment Tool, a form keyed to the six pathways that can help you determine your current baseline of self-care practice. (It is available online; access instructions are e-mailed to all who purchase this book.) You can also use the timetable of your typical day (on p. 33) to assess where you are with your own self-care and to think about how you can infuse moments of self-care into your routine.

A useful resource for any nurse using this book is the HealthyNurse™ website of the American Nurses Association (ANA, 2014) for nurses who want to increase their personal and professional wellness and well-being. ANA defines the healthy nurse "as one who actively focuses on creating and maintaining a balance and synergy of physical, intellectual, emotional, social, spiritual, personal and professional well-being." Self-care is implicit in such a definition. Resources on many of the physical and mental health self-care pathway topics addressed in the sections of this book can be found there. (See also the inside back cover for additional information.)

As a nurse, you may feel that taking care of yourself is something you will do when you "have time," as you are too busy taking care of others. Nurses, as healers, have tremendous influence on creating a healthy and safe environment for patients. As a nurse, the first step is to reflect on your role in the caregiving dynamic. Emulating wellness and disease prevention habits can serve as the seed that germinates change in you, your family, your community, your patients, and eventually the world.

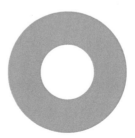

Physical Self-Care Pathway

A healthy body is a guest-chamber for the soul; a sick body is a prison.
—Francis Bacon

Rescue Remedies
for Nurses

Focus on your breath to gain some meditation benefits and stress relief.
Breathe slowly and deeply and be careful not to push any of the stretches further
than feels comfortable.

Play your favorite inspirational music.
Allow the stress to flow through you, without absorbing it, and turn it into positive energy.
Talk to your "accountability buddy", someone you implicitly trust, who will allow you to vent
without judgement and together you agree to actively "let it go...".
Get up, get out, pay a compliment to 5 people in 10 minutes.
Take a brisk walk outside the building, if possible.

Breathe... Breathe... Breathe...

Physical self-care includes proper nutrition, emphasizing disease prevention and management, regular cardiovascular and strength building exercise, adequate sleep and rest, and an understanding of personal self-care routines. Consider consulting your healthcare provider when changing your routines.

Nutrition

Food is information for our genes. The food we eat can be the safest and most powerful form of medicine or the slowest form of poison. Negative stress of any kind, such as infection, poor health choices, difficult life-changing events, personal loss, and emotional trauma all contribute to triggering a damaging inflammatory response in the body. Removing inflammatory triggers is an important intervention to calm down the inflammatory chemicals that are produced when the body perceives it is being "attacked" by foreign entities.

Improving digestion and decreasing inflammation may include dietary modifications, such as the elimination of fried foods, sugars, and any foods that stress an individual's digestive and immune system. Keeping a food journal and then following an elimination diet is helpful in identifying foods that may trigger digestive disorders, food allergies, and immune responses. Removing "triggers" from the diet for a minimum of 21 days can be an important dietary intervention for those with symptoms and possible food sensitivities. Wheat, gluten, lactose, and casein products are the most common foods to eliminate and their elimination may relieve common gastrointestinal problems including constipation, gas and bloating, and irritable bowel syndrome. This is a no-cost intervention that anyone can implement and observe results (Luck, 2009).

Integrating good nutrition into self-care can be a challenge for busy nurses. Begin by asking yourself, "What is one nutrition change that I can make today to improve my health and well-being?" Perhaps you can eliminate refined foods or add whole grains or fiber to your diet. These are simple changes that can make profound differences in your nutritional health.

A prevalence of studies (de Lorgeril & Salen, 2006; Estruch et al., 2013; Hanf & Gonder, 2005; Trichopoulou, Bamia, Lagiou, & Trichopoulos, 2010; Tsivgoulis et al., 2013; Wellman, Kamp, Kirk-Sanchez, & Johnson, 2007) suggest that a Mediterranean diet (a mostly plant-based diet that produces an anti-inflammatory effect) can significantly aid in prevention of cognitive disorders, cardiovascular disease, breast and colon cancers, and stroke. Eating mostly plant-based foods, foods rich in omega-3 fats (such as wild salmon and avocados), snacking on almonds and dark berries, and limiting or eliminating consumption of red meat are all excellent starts towards a healthier diet.

Fiber-rich diets help lower blood cholesterol levels, help stabilize blood sugar levels, and are considered heart-healthy (Park, Subar, Hollenbeck, & Schatzkin, 2011). A fiber-rich diet may reduce risk of infections, respiratory diseases, and heart disease (Park et al., 2011). The U.S. Department of Agriculture (2010) dietary guidelines recommend that at least half of all grains consumed be whole and unrefined. These guidelines recommend 25 grams of fiber per day for women and 28 grams per day for men.

Guidelines for Healthy Choices in Nutrition

As a nurse, you might start your day or night with a high-protein, high-fiber, nutrient-packed meal before work. Nutritional snacks (say, fruit or nuts) or low-fat and high-protein meals (lean meat, Greek-style yogurt) can help you maximize energy and cognitive thinking.

Increase High-Fiber Whole Foods

- Whole grains—Oatmeal, brown rice, quinoa, millet, whole wheat, spelt, barley
- Beans and legumes—Lentils, split peas, garbanzo beans, black beans, hummus, soybeans, and soy foods like tofu and tempeh
- Vegetables—Green, yellow, orange: steamed, raw, or lightly stir-fried
- Nuts and seeds—Sunflower seeds, Brazil nuts, almonds, sesame seeds, pumpkin seeds, nut butters like almond butter, sesame tahini
- Fruits—Local and in season: all berries, papaya, melon, mango, grapefruit

Low-Fat Diet

- Limit meats, especially red meats
- Eliminate sandwich meats (ham, salami, bacon, sausage)
- Increase fish, (being aware of mercury content; see http://www.nrdc.org/health/effects/mercury/guide.asp) as well as chicken and turkey (especially white meat, without skin)
- Use cold-pressed, unprocessed oils such as olive, coconut, or sesame
- Use butter instead of margarine
- Increase omega 3 essential fatty acids (including EPA-DHA), whether as supplements or in organic flax seeds, chia seeds, walnuts, and some fish due to possible mercury content (e.g., canned chunk light tuna is better than canned albacore; see reference above)
- Use low-fat dairy products (as tolerated) or substitutes, such as rice, soy or almond milk
- Bake, broil, steam, or poach

Items to Avoid

- Sugary foods—cookies, soda, candy, jellies, and syrups
- Processed foods—additives, preservatives, artificial colorings, flavorings, corn syrup, and artificial sweeteners like aspartame
- Canned foods—Fresh is best, frozen is next best
- Refined hydrogenated oils—Crisco, palm oil, or cottonseed oil
- Fast foods and junk foods

Other Important Health Tips

- Plan and shop ahead for nutrient-dense, healthy meals
- Prepare several meals ahead of time and freeze/refrigerate so you can bring them to work
- Go to work with at least one healthy snack and meal
- Encourage administration to offer healthy vending machine and cafeteria choices
- Choose organic produce whenever possible as it is free of pesticides
- Drink four to six glasses of liquid daily—spring or filtered water
- Cook and prepare food in cast-iron or stainless steel or glass cookware (avoid aluminum) to prevent chemicals from being leached into your food
- Chew foods slowly and thoroughly
- Read labels and ingredients
- Eat smaller, simpler meals and avoid late-night eating
- Include fiber with each meal.

Source: Luck, 2009

Fats are necessary to optimize healthy lifestyles and prevent chronic illness, but not all fats are equal. For instance, animal fats, hydrogenated fats, and "fake" fats such as margarine create "sludge" and inflammation in arteries. Fats in foods high in omega-3, such as avocados, nuts, seeds, olive oil, and wild-caught salmon help protect your body from internal and external environmental assault. To perform most efficiently and effectively, your body needs "good" fats to keep it running smoothly.

Antioxidants are substances that protect your cells against the effects of free radicals—molecules that are produced when your body breaks down food or when you are exposed to environmental hazards like tobacco smoke and radiation. Free radicals can damage cells and play a role in heart disease, cancer, and other diseases (Lobo, Patil, Phatak, & Chandra, 2010).

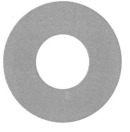

Antioxidants boost immunity and produce an anti-inflammatory effect on the body. Antioxidants are critical for maintaining optimal cellular and systemic health and well-being (Dusting & Triggle, 2005). Antioxidant foods assist with DNA protection, successful repair, and gene expression (Bidlack & Rodriquez, 2012). Foods rich in antioxidants (NIH, 2013) include:

- Beans
- Blueberries
- Broccoli
- Sweet potatoes
- Cranberries

- Blackberries
- Raspberries
- Artichokes
- Prunes
- Kelp (seaweed)

- Turmeric
- Salmon
- Papaya
- Green tea
- Extra virgin olive oil

In a hurry? How about snacking on broccoli or berries? A steamed sweet potato with a drizzle of olive oil makes a great on-the-go lunch. Mix berries in a quick shake with some non-dairy milk and you're off!

Exercise

Regular physical activity that uses large muscle groups—such as walking, running, or swimming—creates cardiovascular changes that increase lung capacity, physical endurance, and heart and skeletal muscle strength. Constant physical activity also prevents the development of coronary artery disease and reduces symptoms in individuals with established cardiovascular disease (Thompson et al., 2003). There is additional evidence that exercise reduces the risk of other chronic diseases, including type two diabetes, osteoporosis, obesity, depression, and breast and colon cancer (Thompson et al., 2003). Various epidemiological studies of occupational and leisure-time physical activity have found a reduced occurrence of coronary artery disease incidents in those who are more physically active and fit. (Thompson et al., 2003)

In 1995, the Centers for Disease Control and Prevention (CDC) and the American College of Sports Medicine (ACSM) recommended that every adult should do 30 minutes or more of moderate-intensity physical activity on most, and preferably all days of the week (Pate et al., 1995). The enduring truth is that there are no shortcuts to physical fitness; the *minimum* amount of exercise is still recommended to be 30 minutes per day (U.S. DHHS, 2008). Consistent exercisers feel more resilient to the challenges of life and can more readily recover from illnesses or injuries. Many people who exercise find their favorite workout activity reduces their stress, enhances their mood, and alleviates physical and mental toxicity.

Inactivity has been shown to have negative effects. The Nurses' Health Study is one of many studies to find a strong link between television watching and obesity (Hu, Li, Colditz, Willet, & Manson, 2003). Researchers followed more than 50,000 middle-aged female nurses for six years, surveying their diet and activity habits. They found that for every two hours the nurses spent watching television each day, they had a 23% higher risk of becoming obese and 14% higher risk of developing diabetes. Interestingly, it didn't matter if the nurses were avid exercisers: the more television they watched, the more likely they were to gain weight or develop diabetes, regardless of their leisure-time activity. Long hours of sitting at work also increased the risk of obesity and diabetes (Hu et al., 2003).

Suggestions for
Physical Self-Care

- Avoid getting dehydrated while working. Use a large personal water container to track the amount of water you drink on a daily basis. Target at least eight ounces every couple of hours, before, during, and after the shift. Make a habit of drinking enough water so that your urine remains clear and pale yellow.

- Talk with your manager about developing of culture of self-care support to help the staff to re-energize and be more productive. This may include creating a type of "serenity room" free of cell phones, interruptions, and food where you can dim the lights, elevate your feet, and close your eyes in a quiet place even for a short period of time.

- Be mindful of your breathing, especially when stressed. Take a few moments each hour to fill up your lungs and slowly exhale. Repeat until you feel your stress level subside.

- Avoid toxic air (smoke, fumes, heavy dust), toxic cleaning solutions, pesticides, personal care products (choose natural products), and noise pollution as much as possible.

- Consider downloading an application on your cell phone that helps track your health goals and use it throughout your shift.

- Sign up for a fitness/yoga class on site or attend a class immediately before/after work. You are much more likely to maintain a regular exercise program in a group setting than alone. Take your accountability buddy!

- Listen to your body. You inherently know if something is "off." Don't ignore signs and symptoms of disease. Make and keep your routine screening appointments.

- Consider wearing a pedometer and walking at least 10,000 steps per day. Perhaps have a contest on your unit with your co-workers.

- Take stretch breaks to re-energize, breathe in new oxygen, and release tension (see examples of stretches on page 8).

- Buddy up with a co-worker to take quick exercise breaks such as stretching or walking around the building, or walking several flights of stairs. Hold each other accountable!

Source: ANA/AONE, 2012

For a busy nurse, the thought of exercising may feel like one more thing to put on your to-do list. However, physically fit nurses have learned to break up the time needed for exercise into chunks that fit their schedules. Even taking the stairs or briskly walking around or within the hospital can help nurses come closer to reaching their daily goals.

A fitness center, either on site or nearby, can be a great place to get a workout. Many hospitals also offer on-site group exercise classes such as yoga, fitness dance, or boot camp. Commit with a buddy to take time each day to exercise. This buddy system will let you hold each other accountable. To minimize excuses, pack workout clothes, a pair of sneakers, and a playlist with your own songs before you head to work. Take a yoga mat to work; during your lunch hour, start a group stretching class in a spare meeting room. Making a routine of stretching often during the day can ease tired muscles, reduce tension, and offer a time of re-energizing. Some stretching examples are shown in Figure 3. These stretching postures do not require any special clothing, shoes, or equipment—just you, your breath, and a few spare minutes.

Sleep and Rest

Nurses need adequate sleep and rest for their self-care; this assures that they are mentally and physically able to think critically and provide the care needed by their patients. In a meta-analysis of the literature of over several hundred studies, Rogers (2008) found there were no positive effects from sleep restriction in healthy adults. Despite the wide range of methodologies, the results are similar: insufficient sleep has been associated with cognitive problems, reduced job performance, increased safety risks, medication errors, mood alterations, and physiological changes. Additionally, depression, irritability, and stress levels increase when sleep is restricted. The meta-analysis also revealed overwhelming evidence that nurses who work longer than 12 consecutive hours or work when they have not obtained sufficient sleep risk negative effects on the health of their patients, themselves, and—if nurses drive home while drowsy—even the general public.

There is also substantial evidence of an increased incidence of diabetes (Ayas et al., 2003; Speigel, Leproult, & VanCauter, 1999) and obesity (Singh, Drake, Roehrs, Hudgel, & Roth, 2005) in sleep-deprived nurses due to significant interference with metabolism and endocrine function. Without enough sleep, cortisol (stress hormone) levels stay high, and the body tries to consistently function in the "fight or flight" mode. As a result, your body loses the ability to regulate hormones effectively (Rogers, 2008).

How much sleep is recommended for adults? The CDC (2013) suggests seven to nine hours of sleep per night. Consider your sleeping environment and make sure it is free of clutter, dark, and quiet. Develop a bedtime routine that triggers your body to prepare for sleep, such as a warm bath or shower, a calming body lotion, soft music or silence, turning off the television, and dimming the lights. Keeping your bed free of computers, cell phones, and any other technology that keeps you in an alert or working state is also very effective.

Your Accountability Buddy and Self-Care

People who succeed often do so with support from others. An accountability buddy is someone who supports you in making sure you meet your self-care commitments, who helps you stay motivated, and who wants to see you succeed—all which will dramatically increase your chances of successfully meeting your goals. While most self-evident with physical self-care, this idea works for all the self-care pathways.

When you choose an accountability buddy (or buddies), think of that person as sharing in your journey. Your accountability buddy may be following a similar journey and the relationship can be mutually beneficial.

Tips for Working with an Accountability Buddy

Write and share your goals. Describe what, how, when, where, and with whom the activity or commitment will take place as well as the potential barriers.

Meet regularly. Decide up front what is reasonable to support mutual goals. Mark your meetings in your calendar and plan everything else around them. In-person meetings are best.

Set time limits. Select a pre-determined amount of time to give an update, ask for help, and make commitments for next steps. Stick to an agenda and be mindful of other people's time.

Respect confidentiality. Respect the confidentiality of each accountability buddy. You or they may speak of personal matters.

Start with a 3-month commitment. Make a commitment longer than a couple of weeks. It helps to know that you are committed to the process.

Start with the end in mind. Start out by discussing what you want out of the relationship by the end of the 3 months (or 6 or 12 months). Exchange emails with your intended goals so you can hold each other accountable.

Offer recognition and praise for small steps that are achieved. Making changes in habits and behavior is difficult and sometimes barriers seem like boulders to prevent success. Recognizing small accomplishments is necessary to prevent throwing in the towel when you or your buddy regress.

If the relationship is not sufficiently supporting you, find another buddy. Don't give up on your goals simply because your buddy is not helpful to you or you feel you are not helping your buddy.

Source: Wieder, 2011.

Mental Self-Care Pathway

One's own self is well hidden from one's own self: of all mines of treasure, one's own is the last to be dug up.
—Friedrich Nietzsche

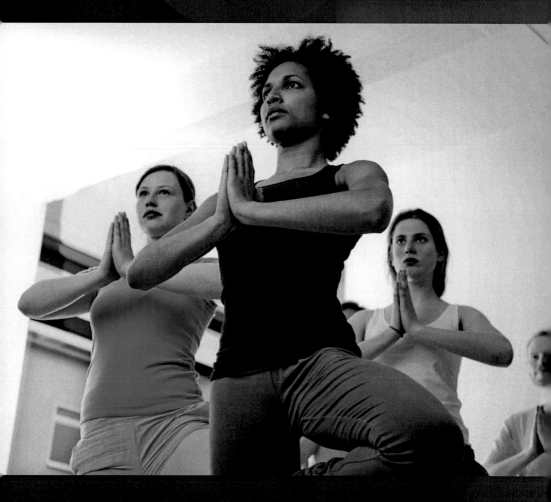

Mental self-care focuses on flexibility, stress-reducing practices, open-mindedness, and constant learning: these are the pillars of a healthy mental environment. Our brains possess extraordinary and untapped potential, but, similar to our muscles, our brains require some "heavy lifting" to grow. (Consider consulting a mental healthcare provider when adopting some of these practices.)

How Stress Harms Your Health

Stress is often described as a feeling of being overwhelmed, worried, or run-down. Stress can affect people of all ages, genders, and circumstances and can lead to both physical and psychological health issues. By definition, stress is any uncomfortable "emotional experience accompanied by predictable biochemical, physiological, and behavioral changes" (Baum, 1990, p. 653). Stress can be beneficial at times, boosting drive and energy to help get through situations like exams or deadlines. However, an extreme amount of stress can have health consequences, adversely affecting the immune, cardiovascular, neuroendocrine, and central nervous systems (Anderson, 1998).

An extraordinary amount of stress can also take a severe emotional toll. While people can overcome minor episodes of stress by tapping into their body's natural defenses to adapt to changing situations, excessive chronic stress, which is constant and persists over an extended period of time, can be psychologically and physically debilitating. Everyday stressors can be controlled with healthy stress management behaviors, but untreated chronic stress can result in serious health conditions, including anxiety, insomnia, muscle pain, high blood pressure, and a weakened immune system (Baum & Polsusnzy, 1999). Research shows that stress can contribute to the development of major illnesses: heart disease, depression, and obesity (Baum & Polsusnzy, 1999). Some studies have even suggested that unhealthy chronic stress management, such as overeating "comfort" foods, has contributed to the growing obesity epidemic (Dallman et al., 2003).

Reducing Stress

Practices that have been helpful in reducing chronic stress include mindfulness, meditation, exercise, positive self-talk, yoga, creative arts, music, and massage.

Mindfulness

Mindfulness has been described as a "moment-to-moment awareness of one's experience without judgment" (Davis & Hayes, 2011, p. 198) and has been shown to ease mental stress. While mindfulness may be attained and cultivated by certain practices, such as meditation, yoga, tai chi, and qigong, it is not equivalent to or synonymous with them (Davis & Hayes, 2012).

Mindfulness practices focus on training attention and voluntarily bringing mental processes under greater control. These processes foster improved mental well-being as well

• 17

as calmness, clarity, and concentration (Walsh & Shapiro, 2006). Mindfulness has been shown to enhance self-insight, morality, intuition, and fear modulation—all functions associated with the brain's middle prefrontal lobe, which we utilize in critical thinking. Evidence also suggests that mindfulness meditation has numerous health benefits, including increased immune functioning (Davidson et al., 2003). Other benefits of mindfulness practice include:

- **Reduced rumination** (Chambers, Lo, & Allen, 2008)
- **Stress reduction** (Hoffman, Sawyer, Witt, & Oh, 2010)
- **Boosts to working memory** (Jha, Stanley, Kiyonaga, Wong, & Gelfand, 2010)
- **Focus** (Moore & Malinowski, 2009)
- **Less emotional reactivity** (Ortner, Kilner, & Zelazo, 2007)
- **More cognitive flexibility** (Siegel, 2007)
- **More adaptive responses to stressful or negative situations** (Cahn & Polich, 2006; Davidson et al., 2003)
- **Relationship satisfaction** (Barnes, Brown, Krusemark, Campbell, & Rogge, 2007)

Even practicing mindfulness for a period of two weeks has been shown to create changes in the brain (Hanson, 2009). Neurons that fire together, wire together. These new patterns of thought can actually change the physiology of our brains, training us to become more alert to good information.

How is mindfulness practiced? When you notice a positive detail in yourself or someone else, or in your environment, savor it for at least ten seconds. Most of these observations will be as simple as "the sun is shining" or "this coffee tastes good," but if you do this a handful of times each day, you'll feel an emotional shift.

Discovering mindfulness techniques and routinely practicing stress reduction are great ways to keep up with the demand and intensity of our lives. Practicing mindfulness helps to increase awareness. Noise pollution in the forms of violent television, drama-filled newscasts, and constant chatter are absorbed into our brains on a daily basis if we aren't vigilant about applying limits or trauma filters.

Meditation

Lazar et al. (2000) studied meditation and brain activation and found that meditation activates certain neural structures pertaining to attention and arousal/autonomic control; these neural structures are related to anxiety and emotional distress. Therefore, simply taking 10 minutes a day to find stillness, allow the mind to quiet and calm, and focus on deep breathing offers an opportunity to push your reset button. The power of this relaxation response and the concurrent release of endorphins has a calming effect on the mind, body, and spirit. This practice, if done on a regular basis, can create new "grooves" in the brain and become the new default route, bypassing the fight or flight response often triggered by stress (Lazar et al., 2000).

Davidson et al. (2003) led a study comparing a meditation group with a non-meditation group. Brain electrical activity was measured before, immediately after, and four months after an eight-week training program in mindfulness meditation ($N = 41$). The meditation group showed a significant increase in activation of left-side anterior electrical activity, a part of the brain that has previously been associated with positive affect. The findings in this study show that a short mindfulness meditation program can create apparent positive changes in the brain.

One form of mantra meditation is transcendental meditation (TM). Benson (1985) found that the mantra meditation in TM evoked a relaxation response and went on to modify the Sanskrit words of the mantra. He then experimented with simple, positive statements devoid of any spiritual implications and demonstrated that a relaxation response could be evoked by any combination of repetitive, simple, positive statements.

Transcendental meditation is very simple. "A trained instructor gives you a secret word or sound or phrase—a mantra—that you promise not to divulge. This sound is allegedly chosen to suit the individual and is to be silently 'perceived.' The meditator receives the mantra from his teacher and then repeats it mentally over and over again while sitting in a comfortable position. Meditators are told to assume a passive attitude and if other thoughts come into mind to disregard them, going back to the mantra. Practitioners are advised to meditate twenty minutes in the morning, usually before breakfast, and twenty minutes in the evening, usually before dinner." (Benson, 2000, p. 63).

Another way to calm your mind and body is "Let Go" practice (Schaub & Schaub, 2013). It triggers a good response because of its simplicity and the ability to do it anywhere at any time, perhaps before or during a difficult conversation, after a critical incident, or when you need to release tension. The steps include:

- Close or lower your eyes and let your shoulders drop.
- Now say a three-word phrase in your mind. The first word in the phrase is your first name, and the next two words are "let go." Repeat this over and over again in your mind, taking your time.
- You can link the three-word phrase to your in-breath, your out-breath, or not link it to your breath at all. Experiment to find the way you like best.
- Continue saying your first name, followed by "let go," repeating it over and over again in your mind.
- Wait two minutes and then say, "And now let go of the practice and turn your attention toward noticing how you are."
- Wait 30 seconds and then say, "And when you feel ready, at your own pace, begin to come back to the room and open your eyes."

Exercise and Stress

The effects of exercise on stress are significant. Physical activity increases your body's production of feel-good endorphins, a type of neurotransmitter in the brain, and helps in treating mild forms of depression and anxiety (Fox, 1999). Taking one small step to reduce your stress and improve your emotional health, such as going on a daily walk, can have a beneficial effect. Being active is a powerful change you can make to manage stress.

Self-Talk and Stress

Self-talk is another key element of the mental self-care pathway, but self-talk can be negative or positive. Negative self-talk is any conversation with yourself that undermines your ability to reach your highest potential—a conversation in which you start to believe that you are unable or unworthy. The loop of self-talk and subsequent anxiety has been referred to as the "monkey mind" and is not always kind and encouraging (Smith, 2012). Monkey-mind chatter has been described as easily distracting, fearful, or the voice of the "what-ifs." Your monkey mind could be the voice of the teacher who told you that you were terrible at math when you are trying to calculate a medication dose, or the voice of a sibling who criticized your ability to select the right outfit when you are deciding what to wear for an important talk in front of your peers. It's the self-doubt we experience when we ruminate over a difficult situation.

Learning to translate negative self-talk into positive self-talk is an extremely effective strategy to ease mental stress. Your positive self-talk may sound like this: "I'm really proud of you and how you make a positive difference in the lives of others!"; "I see the goodness and compassion in all you do!"; "I love the uniqueness of you!"; or "You rock!"

The power of positive self-talk is astounding! You may find it helpful to post positive affirmations in your living space. Give yourself a boost by offering a bit of positive self-talk whenever you catch a glimpse of yourself in a mirror or window.

Yoga

The practice of yoga has been studied in relation to many risk factors for chronic disease states. Yang (2007), in a review of articles, found that yoga interventions were generally effective in reducing body weight, blood pressure, glucose level, and high cholesterol. However, only a few studies examined long-term adherence. Other physical benefits of yoga (Nevins, 2013) include:

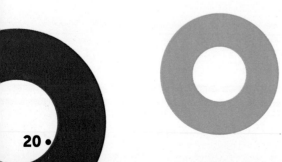
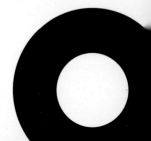

- Increased flexibility;
- Increased muscle strength and tone;
- Improved respiration, energy, and vitality;
- The maintenance of a balanced metabolism;
- Weight reduction;
- Cardiac and circulatory health;
- Improved athletic performance; and
- Protection from injury.

Aside from the array of physical benefits, another great benefit of yoga is how it helps people manage stress. There are many ways in which stress reveals itself, including neck and back pain, headaches, insomnia, and a general inability to concentrate; by helping with stress-management techniques, yoga can reduce some of these symptoms. People who practice yoga feel more able to handle the inconsistencies of life. Unlike more traditional forms of exercise, the way yoga incorporates meditation and breathing helps individuals integrate these practices into their daily lives to improve their mental and spiritual well-being.

For over 5,000 years, yoga has evolved, morphed with other exercise formats, and become a mainstream form of exercise. Visit a yoga studio today and you will see a reflection of a modern society, with many different yoga styles (over 100) and formats. There are abundant articles and journals, as well as evidence-based research that support the practice of yoga as a way to self-heal. Even with various styles of yoga, most sessions are typically comprised of breathing exercises, meditation, and assuming postures (sometimes called *asanas* or poses) that stretch and flex various muscle groups. Regular practice of all three parts of this yoga structure produces a more focused mind and a strong, capable body.

Examples of Proactive Self-Care Language

- Thank you for considering me for this project. It sounds very exciting! Could we please meet to review my current responsibilities? I would like to be able to give my best efforts to this new idea and feel that some of my other projects might be better served by someone else at this time.
- I'm in time-out!
- I would love to serve on that committee but I don't have the time or energy right now to do it justice.
- I'm taking a me day and will not be available (turn off cell phone).

Tai Chi

Tai chi is an ancient Chinese tradition that, today, is practiced as a graceful form of exercise. It involves a series of movements performed in a slow, focused manner, attaching breath with movement. Tai chi is a self-paced system of gentle physical exercise and stretching. Each posture flows into the next without pause, ensuring that the body is in constant motion. It is sometimes referred to as a gentle moving meditation that aids in reduction of stress and the promotion of psychological well-being (Wang et al., 2010), as well as other health benefits (Jahnke et al., 2010; Tai Chi Research, 2014.). Tai chi classes are available in most communities or health centers.

Getting lost in a favorite book, saying "no" to overcommitting, listening to inspirational music, painting, participating in favorite hobbies, singing, getting massages or pedicures, or whatever meets your definition of "aahhh..." are all ways of reducing stress. Relaxing the mind and creating an inner calm are all central to self-care.

Routines and rhythms allow you to relax, let go of resistance, and settle into a place of effortless mental comfort. Whatever your choice of stress reduction, you must be proactive and consistent until it becomes a habit that is part of your daily life. Exploring what works best for you is part of your unique self-care journey.

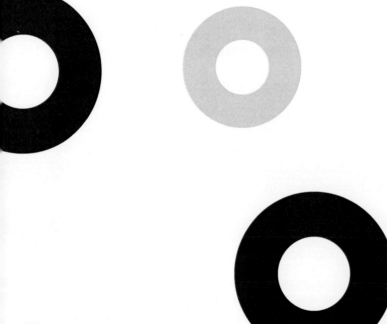

Suggestions for Mental Self-Care

- Start each day with a positive affirmation; expect a good day.
- Post short, positive notes to yourself in highly visible areas around your home or personal workspace.
- Write in a gratitude journal. Or write a note when you are grateful for something and put it in a gratitude jar. When you are feeling down, pull a few out to shift your attitude.
- Eliminate any appointments that are not necessary.
- Each day, practice kind, supportive self-talk in the mirror.
- Sign up for positive affirmations on your email or cell phone.
- Say "no" without feeling guilty. Take time to think before overcommitting.
- De-clutter one room, even one drawer at a time. Invite a friend over to help with donating old or unused items.
- Spend 10 minutes alone each day to bring yourself into the present moment. Meditate, deeply breathe, practice the "Let Go" technique, or listen to relaxing music. Let your mind be thoughtless, settling into the feeling of calm.
- Celebrate accomplishments! Collect mementoes that remind you of your achievements or write them on the notes posted around you.
- Disconnect from your computer, cell phone, and/or pager once a day. Don't answer or expect a response immediately. Never allow your computer or cell phone in bed with you!
- Check out the latest apps available for stress reduction practice and download them onto your phone.
- Surround your space with words/phrases, cartoons, or images that encourage and support you.
- Schedule a weekly massage (check out massage schools for reasonable fees).
- Schedule whatever makes you feel pampered and stick to it. You are creating a habit.
- Accept compliments with a simple "thank you!" Give compliments often.
- Savor good moods, positive emotions, and warm memories to become more aware of opportunities in everyday life to nurture yourself.

Other Self-Care Pathways

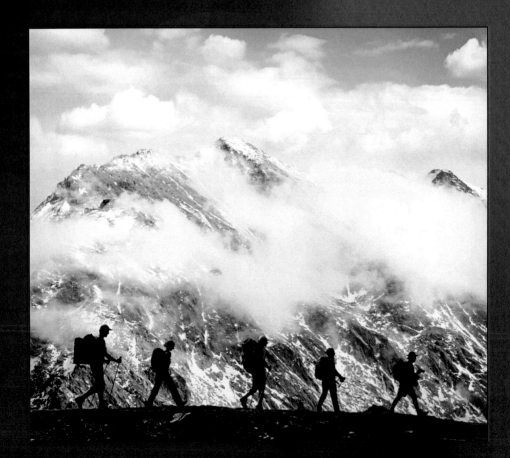

Emotional Self-Care

A sad soul can kill you quicker than a germ.

—John Steinbeck

Emotions are a dominant part of the human condition. We engage in constant dialogue within ourselves; how we feel, perceive, and respond is regulated by our emotional state. Past joys, hurts, and traumatic events all contribute to our emotional health, yet we can choose to release toxic feelings that hold us back or no longer serve us well. Emotional baggage can be exhausting. Identifying where unresolved emotional pain is eroding your self-care is freeing for both you and those around you.

Fredrickson (2009), Csikszentmihalyi (1990), and Seligman (2002) are part of what is known as the positive psychology movement and have aided in focusing attention on what is satisfying, energizing, hopeful, resilient, and happy. They have discovered that happiness is a state you can practice and cultivate, and that it depends on your choices, attitudes, and thoughts.

The research on positive psychology suggests that every person has a baseline for happiness. Positive and negative life events will affect your baseline, but over time you have a tendency to return to about the same level of happiness. Your baseline depends on your temperament and genetics as well as your fundamental beliefs.

Your belief system becomes a habit of your thinking, but sometimes you incorporate inaccurate thinking patterns: if you think you are not as good as other people, you are sad; if you think you will lose social standing, you are embarrassed. People who acquire self-knowledge about these inaccurate beliefs and feelings can permanently raise their baseline of happiness. The more you recognize your thinking patterns and beliefs, the more you can understand inaccuracies and change your ways of thinking.

The ability to see events and situations from a positive perspective serves to strengthen resilience. Positive people are more flexible and have a noticeable "bounce back" factor; they also have self-nurturing coping skills. It's not that positive people don't experience grief and suffering; they simply *choose* to move forward instead of wallowing in sadness. Overall, positive people *choose* to live in a state of well-being.

Tim Kasser, an expert in the study of well-being, links well-being to the fulfillment of four psychological needs: safety and security, competence, connection to other people, and autonomy or freedom (Kasser & Sheldon, 2001). It is imperative to happiness to find a balance between pleasure and meaning.

According to Csikszentmihalyi (1990), a critical ingredient to a happy life is "flow," occasions when you are so focused in an activity that you become absorbed and even lose track of time. While you are in the flow, you are not aware of being happy, because happiness would distract you from what you are

Suggestions for Emotional Self-Care

- Be aware of your instinctive emotional responses and start consciously challenging the negative thoughts and restricting belief systems that underlie them.

- Create a self-calming or hopeful mental mantra, e.g., "This, too, shall pass" or "I get to choose my responses."

- Ask for help before you feel overwhelmed. Delegate and let it be. Know the delegatee may not complete the task perfectly, but it's not worth your extra stress.

- List the times you have experienced "flow." When do you lose track of time? What were you doing? Can you start adding those activities to your schedule and budget?

- What kinds of hobbies do you enjoy? Create opportunities to learn something new or expand your abilities in different areas of your life.

- Put effort into doing something considerate, loving, and generous for others daily—random acts of kindness for which you don't get recognition or payment. Grasp every opportunity to do the right thing and to express gratitude for kindnesses you receive. Also try and get involved with an organization that doesn't just want your money, but also asks for some face-to-face time and effort.

- Seek professional assistance if you feel you are hanging onto old emotional baggage. Letting go of past hurts allows you to be free to cultivate positive emotions.

- Start journaling about how you feel. Writing down emotions allows you to let go, release negativity, and move on. If you feel you need professional help, seek it.

- Spend time with your companion pets. Allow yourself to feel their love for you.

- Take a walk outside. With each step, visualize stress, negativity and anxiety literally falling away from your body.

- Protect your sensitivity by being aware of surroundings such as lighting, pictures, sounds, and color. Create a peaceful environment in your home, especially in your bedroom. Little details matter.

- Learn to transition your mood as you are traveling to and from work by listening to music, or choosing silence instead. Don't feel compelled to fill each minute of time. Perhaps take a different route to work or stop by a park or coffee shop.

- Have a safe friend or colleague to vent to who will simply listen and agree to let it go.

doing. But after you have finished and look back, you recognize your happiness when you applied yourself fully to the task at hand. Csikszentmihalyi discovered that "flow" can occur regardless of activity. Someone can cultivate flow whether organizing paint cans or preparing a seminal speech at work. Achieving the state of flow requires being present, having a problem-solving attitude, and having the conviction you are going to give it your best. Try shifting your mindset from "here is another stupid task I have to do" to "I am going to do it as well as possible."

Fundamental to positive psychology is the belief that happiness is found not only through individual thoughts and behaviors, but also by engaging in a wider purpose and contributing to the wellness of others. Embracing virtues, acting on them, and enjoying their rewards are critical behaviors for bettering emotional health. Many people find that volunteering for a cause they strongly believe in continually feeds their emotional needs, even though they may only participate occasionally. It's the emotional connectedness—a key element of emotional self-care—that matters. For other ideas on emotional self-care, see the sidebar on this/the next page.

Spiritual Self-Care

> *People say that what we're all seeking is a meaning for life. I don't think that's what we're really seeking. I think that what we're seeking is an experience of being alive.*
>
> —Joseph Campbell

Spiritual self-care is a reflection of your belief in a higher power that connects you with the universe. Your beliefs might or might not be rooted in organized religion, but the spirit reflected is uniquely yours. Your beliefs shape your perceptions of your world and so serve to either nurture your soul or deplete your spirit. The power of spirituality can be felt every day and is good for your health. Spiritual believers are physically healthier, lead healthier lifestyles, and require fewer health services, adding 7 to 14 years to life expectancy (Hummer, Rogers, Nam, & Ellison, 1999).

What makes you feel most connected with your spiritual beliefs? When do you feel the most alive? Perhaps your spiritual self-care involves contributing to a cause, participating in a spiritual ceremony, taking a nature walk, or visiting an art museum. For example, art allows us to further investigate the subliminal layers of meaning that we experience in our everyday lives. Sometimes art shows us what is felt, but is hard to put into words.

For some, organized religious practices serve to bring connection to a higher power. Worship in the form of prayer, meditation, music, singing, and group leadership often defines spiritual self-care. Others find connectedness in the practice of yoga, tai chi, or creative outlets such as dance and writing. Knowing what activities and practices feed your spirit and make you feel a loving presence is the key to spiritual self-care.

Suggestions for Spiritual Self-Care

- Collect a symbol, artifact, or mandala that reflects your spiritual beliefs and place it in a highly visible area in your home.
- Consider a daily spiritual practice such as devotional reading, meditation, or prayer. If being in nature is part of what feeds you, schedule that time and drink it in!
- If an organized religion is part of your spiritual practice, participate in ways of worship such as singing in the choir, leading study groups, and making outreach contacts.
- Write down your core values and develop activities that support, strengthen, and reflect those values.
- Consider a pilgrimage to deepen your connection with your beliefs and/or higher purpose.
- Volunteer your time and talent to a cause that supports a core value.
- Read poetry or inspirational stories or listen to music that resonates with your spirituality.
- Forgive often and with grace to keep your heart open.

Your spiritual journey can be one of being both a teacher and a student. As a nurse, the gravity of suffering and illness can often challenge your spiritual beliefs. Yet you also get to see the entire cycle of life in all its forms. Proactively filling up your soul serves to keep your heart open to the abundance of life and your calling to be a healer.

Relationship Self-Care

Those who have a hard time receiving attract those who have a hard time giving.

—Christiane Northrup

The profound impact of who we choose (or do not choose) to spend our lives with cannot be overstated. Our lives are affected, either positively or negatively, by the quality of our relationships, starting with the one you have with yourself. Your relationship with yourself is the foundation from which all others flow.

What we think of ourselves, how we treat ourselves, and how we respect ourselves are the foundational elements essential in the

Suggestions for Relationship Self-Care

- Set aside some time every day to connect with important people in your life. Create weekly or other regular customs that give you an opportunity to interact with others in a meaningful way.
- Limit exposure to people who drain your energy and leave you feeling exhausted. If possible, politely decline to participate in activities where those people will be; if not possible, visualize a bubble surrounding you that lets their negative energy bounce off of you.
- Be mindful of the words you use with others and the impact they may have.
- Ramp up your time with people who pump you up, believe in your dreams, and want the absolute best for you.
- Choose a mentor for yourself and become a mentor to another.
- Never miss an opportunity to tell those you love how much they mean to you.
- Weed the toxic people from your garden of relationships.
- Always speak your truth with grace and love.
- Be a good friend and companion. Be fully present and limit interruptions such as phone conversations and texting. Request that the people you are with do the same.

creation of supporting, loving, compassionate, and long-lasting relationships. If we don't love ourselves, how can we expect others to? If we aren't clear about who we are and what we want in our lives, how can we possibly expect others to know?

The relationship pathway of self-care, although sometimes elusive, is fundamental to building a purpose-driven life. When we have the courage to be authentic and speak truthfully, we attract others who reflect the same values and want the best life for us. Conversely, if we allow another person to put our compass in their pocket, we lose our life's footing. The quality of the relationship you have with yourself depends on whether you listen to your small, inner voice of intuition and trust your gut feelings; doing this will help you continue your personal journey to shine your light, feeling the full reflection of your warmth.

Self-care may be challenged when dealing with toxic people or toxic relationships. As nurses, we are willing to help, fix, or support others, sometimes at the expense of our own health. Relationships either add to or subtract from your life and must be a two-way street to be fulfilling. To live your healthiest life, sometimes it becomes necessary to weed out toxic people from your "garden" of relationships, letting go of the struggle and allowing yourself to move on.

Toxic people can come in many forms. Do you feel on edge or guarded around certain individuals? Do you know people who dump their drama, chronic anger, and unresolved issues at your feet? Do you interact with people who disrespect you or put you down? As we teach others how to treat us, we should emulate self-respect, communication, and healthy support of each other.

Relationships can make you uncomfortable and can mirror some of your own faults and insecurities. The qualities you dislike in others often reflect qualities in yourself that you dislike. Want to change your quality of relationships? First change the relationship you have with yourself.

Be mindful of evolving relationship patterns that tend to have a negative outcome. Those who sincerely care about you will welcome your need to clarify, define, and explore ways to deepen connections.

The practices of self-care have also been proven to be of great support in developing teamwork. A recent study (N = 20 care units) identified that self-care had a significant relationship involving teamwork with nurses (r = .519, p < .019) (Hozak & Brennan, 2012). Nurses who are positive, passionate about caring, and practice self-nurturing behaviors tend to be supportive team members. The energy in a team of healthy nurses has the ability to transform culture.

Christakis and Fowler (2007) followed 12,067 subjects from the Framingham Heart Study over the course of 32 years. A person's chance of becoming obese increased by 57% if a friend became obese. The type of friendship is also important. Between mutual friends, a subject's risk of obesity increased by a whopping 171% if the friend became obese. It seems that, among friendship groups, social modeling may play a significant role in the spread of obesity (Herman, Roth, & Polivy, 2003; Hetherington, 2007; Hetherington, Anderson, Norton, & Newson, 2006). This research has clear implications for choosing a positive relationship pathway in terms of self-care and is a prime example of how pathways intersect.

Choice Self-Care Pathway

There is no need to go to India or anywhere else to find peace. You will find that deep place of silence right in your room, your garden or even your bathtub.

—Elisabeth Kubler-Ross

Your life right now, in this moment, is like a snapshot of every single choice you have made throughout your lifetime, both "good" and "not so good." When you make choices from self-compassion, and the choices are in line with your core values, neither self-sacrifice nor self-flagellation has a place. Choosing to create a life of improved self-care takes a little effort, but with each new thought and action towards your goals, you will feel the burden lighten, drama subside, and you will have a renewed sense of freedom. The key is to keep doing the practices you choose until they become ingrained habits and you form a self-motivating routine.

Suggestions for Choice Self-Care

- Recycle, reuse, and donate.
- Consider hiring a house cleaner or someone to help with outdoor chores once a month. Your time is valuable. How much are you worth?
- Refuse to listen to a rumor or nasty gossip. Speak up and don't feed drama.
- Sign up to receive current healthy lifestyle information from reputable websites. Educate yourself and your community on new information.
- Choose to be an example of wellness and emulate healthy habits.
- Choose an accountability buddy!

There is nothing more effective in showing you where you are stuck, where you need to grow, and what lessons you need to learn than the obstacles that cross your path. Obstacles are the ultimate teachers; they allow you to reset your path. You can choose to resist and push against obstacles more forcefully, exhausting yourself, or you can choose to take a step back, observe, process, and carefully choose your next step. Doing nothing and being neutral is also a choice. When you don't know what path to choose, allowing yourself to be uncomfortable and uneasy will improve your resilience to overcome future hurdles and difficulty down the road. The pathway of choice is inclusive of all of other pathways, and represents your plan to practice self-care as a lifestyle. Choice self-care embodies a way of living, being, and behaving.

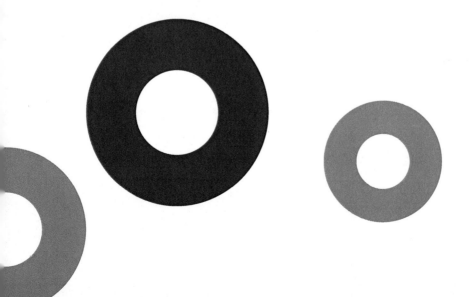

Self-Care and You:
A Lifelong Journey

Healing is a lifelong journey into wholeness.
Becoming healed involves learning to trust life.
—Barbara Dossey

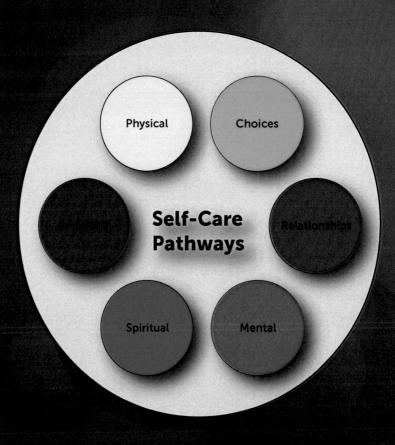

As a professional registered nurse, you are part of a trusted profession that includes over three million individuals. The potential to affect the health of the United States and the world is within reach. You have an opportunity to profoundly influence your family and friends as well as to contribute to the health and wellness of your community by personally choosing a healthy lifestyle.

Your practice of self-care is a lifelong journey, one of many stages and steps along the pathways detailed in these pages. It can be pursued on your own or with others throughout your day; a suggested sequence is shown in the checklist below. Also consider using the Self-Care Assessment Tool (available online as noted on pg. 7) along your way to update your awareness of your self-care practice baseline. Use such resources and the opportunities they provide to reflect how you are caring for yourself and, if needed, make the changes necessary to optimize your quality of life.

You represent the heart and soul of healing and compassion. Take the time to routinely fuel the flame that keeps your passion for nursing burning bright. Contribute to solutions and commit to do your part to create healthy change. The lifestyle you cultivate—both in self-care and in care for others—has the power to heal the world. You hold the key!

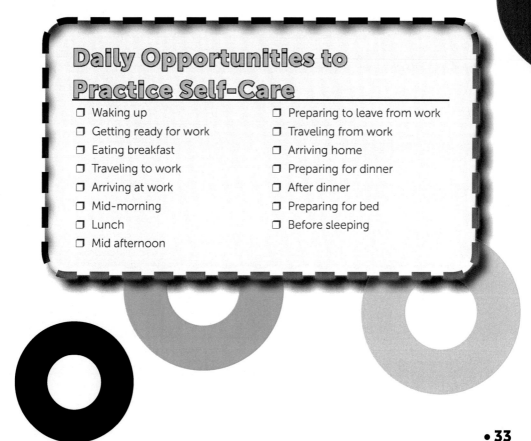

Daily Opportunities to Practice Self-Care

- ❒ Waking up
- ❒ Getting ready for work
- ❒ Eating breakfast
- ❒ Traveling to work
- ❒ Arriving at work
- ❒ Mid-morning
- ❒ Lunch
- ❒ Mid afternoon
- ❒ Preparing to leave from work
- ❒ Traveling from work
- ❒ Arriving home
- ❒ Preparing for dinner
- ❒ After dinner
- ❒ Preparing for bed
- ❒ Before sleeping

Bibliography

Absolon, P., & Krueger, C. (2009). Compassion fatigue nursing support group in ambulatory care gynecology/oncology nursing. *Journal of Gynecologic Oncology Nursing*, 19(1), 16–19.

American Nurses Association. (2014). HealthyNurse™. Retrieved from http://www.nursingworld.org/MainMenuCategories/WorkplaceSafety/Healthy-Nurse

American Nurses Association. (2001). *Code of Ethics for Nurses with interpretive statements.* Silver Spring, MD: Nursesbooks.org.

Anderson, N. B. (1998). Levels of analysis in health science: A framework for integrating sociobehavioral and biomedical research. *Annals of the New York Academy of Sciences*, 840, 563–576.

Ayas, N., White, D. P., Al-Delaimy, W. K., Manson, J. E., Stampfer, M. J., Speizer, F. E., Patel, S., & Hu, F. B. (2003). A prospective study of self-reported sleep duration and incidence of diabetes in women. *Diabetes Care,* 26(2), 380–384.

Aycock, N., & Boyle, D. (2009). Interventions to manage compassion fatigue in oncology nursing. *Clinical Journal of Oncology Nursing,* 13, 183–191.

Barnes, S., Brown, K. W., Krusemark, E., Campbell, W. K., & Rogge, R. D. (2007). The role of mindfulness in romantic relationship satisfaction and responses to relationship stress. *Journal of Marital and Family Therapy*, 33, 482–500. doi:10.1111/j.1752–0606.2007.00033.x

Baum, A. (1990). Stress, intrusive imagery, and chronic distress. *Health Psychology*, 6, 653–675.

Baum, A., & Polsusnzy, D. (1999). Health psychology: Mapping biobehavioral contributions to health and illness. *Annual Review of Psychology*, 50, 137–163.

Benson, H. (2000). *The relaxation response.* New York: Harper Collins.

Benson, H. (1985). *Beyond the relaxation response.* Berkley, CA: Penguin.

Bidlack, W., & Rodriguez, R. (2012). *Nutritional genomics: The impact of dietary regulation of gene function on human disease.* Boca Raton, FL: Taylor and Francis Group, LLC.

Bland, J. (2012, February 9). *Clinical implications of epigenetics.* Keynote address, Integrative Healthcare Symposium, New York.

Cahn, B. R., & Polich, J. (2006). Meditation states and traits: EEG, ERP, and neuroimaging studies. *Psychological Bulletin*, 132, 180–211. doi:10.1037/0033–2909.132.2.180

Centers for Disease Control and Prevention (CDC). (2013). *Sleep disorders: How much sleep do I need?* Atlanta, GA. Retrieved from http://www.cdc.gov/sleep/about_sleep/how_much_sleep.htm

Chambers, R., Lo, B. C. Y., & Allen, N. B. (2008). The impact of intensive mindfulness training on attentional control, cognitive style, and affect. *Cognitive Therapy and Research*, 32, 303–322. doi:10.1007/s10608-007-9119-0

Christakis, N. A., & Fowler, J. H. (2007). The spread of obesity in a large social network over 32 years. *New England Journal of Medicine,* 357, 370–379.

Csikszentmihalyi, M. (1990). *Flow.* New York: Harper and Row.

Dallman, M., Pecoraro, N., Akana, S., la Fleur, S., Gomez, F., Houshyar, H., ... Manalo, S. (2003). Chronic stress and obesity: A new view of 'comfort food.' *Proceedings of the National Academy of Sciences,* 100, 11696–11701.

Davidson, R. J., Kabat-Zinn, J., Schumacher, J., Rosenkranz, M., Muller, D., Santorelli, S. F., ...Sheridan, J. F. (2003). Alterations in brain and immune function produced by mindfulness meditation. *Psychosomatic Medicine,* 66, 149–152. doi:10.1097/01. psy.0000116716.19848.65

Davis, D., & Hayes, J., (2011). What are the benefits of mindfulness? A practice review of psychotherapy related research. *Psychotherapy,* 48(2), 198–208.

de Lorgeril, M., & Salen, P. (2006). The Mediterranean diet in secondary prevention of coronary heart disease. *Clinical Investigative Medicine,* 3, 154–158.

Dossey, B. (2012). Integral, integrative, and holistic—local to global. In B. Dossey & L. Keegan, *Holistic nursing: A handbook for practice* (p. 157–165). Sudbury, MA: Jones and Bartlett Publishers.

Dossey, B. M., & Keegan, L. (2009). *Holistic nursing: A handbook for practice.* Sudbury, MA: Jones and Bartlett Publishers.

Dusting, J., & Triggle, C. (2005). Are we overoxidized? Oxidative stress, cardiovascular disease, and the future of intervention studies with antioxidants. *Vascular Health Risk Management,* 1(2), 93–97.

Estruch, R., Ros, E., Salas-Salvadó, J., Covas, M. I., Corella, D., Arós, F., ... Martínez-González, M. A. (2013). Primary prevention of cardiovascular disease with a Mediterranean diet. *New England Journal of Medicine,* 368, 1279–1290. doi: 10.1056/NEJMoa1200303

Figley, C. (2002). Compassion fatigue: Psychotherapists' chronic lack of self care. *Journal of Clinical Psychology,* 58(11), 1433–1441.

Fox, K. R. (1999). The influence of physical activity on mental well-being. *Public Health Nutrition,* 2, 411–418.

Fredrickson, B., (2009) *Positivity.* New York: Crown Publishing.

Gould, J. E. (2005). Compassion fatigue: An expert interview with Charles R. Figley, MS, PhD. *Medscape News.* Retrieved from: www.medscape.comlviewarticlel513615.

Hanf, V., & Gonder, U. (2005). Nutrition and primary prevention of breast cancer: foods, nutrients and breast cancer risk. *European Journal of Obstetrical, Gynecology, and Reproductive Biology,* 123(2), 139–149.

Hanson, R. (2009). *Buddha's brain: The practical neuroscience of happiness, love and wisdom.* Oakland, CA: New Harbinger Publications.

Herman, C. P., Roth, D. A., & Polivy, J. (2003). Effects of the presence of others on food intake: A normative interpretation. *Psychological Bulletin,* 129, 873–886.

Hetherington, M. M. (2007). Cues to overeat: Psychological factors influencing over-consumption. *Proceedings of the Nutrition Society,* 66, 113–123.

Hetherington, M. M., Anderson, A. S., Norton, G. N. M., & Newson, L. (2006). Situational effects on meal intake: A comparison of eating alone and eating with others. *Physiology and Behavior,* 88, 498–505.

Hoffman, S. G., Sawyer, A. T., Witt, A. A., & Oh, D. (2010). The effect of mindfulness-based therapy on anxiety and depression: A meta-analytic review. *Journal of Consulting and Clinical Psychology,* 78, 169–183. doi:10.1037/a0018555

Hooper, C., Craig, J., Janvrin, D. R., Wetsel, M. A., & Reimels, E. (2010). Compassion satisfaction, burnout, and compassion fatigue among emergency nurses compared with nurses in other selected inpatient specialties. *Journal of Emergency Nursing, 36*(5), 420–427.

Hozak, M. A., & Brennan, M. (2012). Caring at the core: Maximizing the likelihood that a caring moment will occur. In J. Nelson & J. Watson, (Eds.), *Measuring caring: A compilation of international research on caritas as healing intervention* (p. 195–224). New York: Springer.

Hu, F. B., Li, T. Y., Colditz, G., Willett, W., & Manson, J. (2003). Television watching and other sedentary behaviors in relation to risk of obesity and type 2 diabetes mellitus in women. *Journal of the American Medical Association 289*, 1785–1791.

Hummer, R., Rogers, R., Nam, C., & Ellison, C. G. (1999). Religious involvement and U. S. adult mortality. *Demography, 36*, 273–285.

Hyman, M. A., Ornish, D., & Roizen, M. (2009). Life style medicine: Treating the causes of disease. *Alternative Therapies, 15*(6), 12–14.

Jahnke, R., Larkey, L., Rogers, C., Etnier, J. & Lin, F. (2010) A comprehensive review of health benefits of Qigong and Tai Chi. *American Journal of Health Promotion, 24*(6): e1–e25. (July/August.) doi: http://dx.doi.org/10.4278/ajhp.081013-LIT-248. Retrieved from http://www.ncbi.nlm.nih.gov/pmc/articles/PMC3085832/

Jha, A. P., Stanley, E. A., Kiyonaga, A., Wong, L., & Gelfand, L. (2010). Examining the protective effects of mindfulness training on working memory capacity and affective experience. *Emotion, 10*, 54–64. doi:10.1037/a0018438.

Johnson, R. W. (2010). *Chronic care: Making the case for ongoing care*. Princeton, NJ: Robert Wood Johnson Foundation. Retrieved from www.rwjf.org/pr/product.jsp.

Johnson, S. (2012). A U.S. study of nurses' self-care and compassion fatigue using Watson's concepts of caritas. In J. Nelson & J. Watson (Eds.), *Measuring caring: A compilation of international research on caritas as healing intervention* (p. 413–420). New York: Springer.

Kasser, T. & Sheldon., K. (2001). Goals, congruence, and positive well-being: New empirical support for humanistic theories. *Journal of Humanistic Psychology, 41*, 30–50.

Kearney, M. K., Weininger, R. B., Vachon, M. L., Harrison, R. L., & Mount, B. M. (2009). Self-care of physicians caring for patients at the end of life. *Journal of the American Medical Association*, 301(11), 1155–1164.

Keegan, L. & Dossey, B. (2004) Self-care: a program to improve your life, Holistic Nursing Consultants. In B. Dossey & L. Keegan, *Holistic nursing: A handbook for practice* (p.159–165). Sudbury, MA: Jones and Bartlett.

Lazar, S. W., Bush, G., Gollub, R. L., Fricchione, G. L., Khalsa, G., & Benson, H. (2000). Functional brain mapping of the relaxation response and meditation. *Neuroreport*, 11(7), 1581–1585.

Lobo, V., Patil, A., Phatak, A., & Chandra, N. (2010). Free radicals, antioxidants, and functional foods: Impact on human health. *Pharmacognosy Review, 4*(8), 118–126. doi: 10.4103/0973-7847.70902

Luck, S. (2009). Nutrition. In B. M. Dossey & L. Keegan, (Eds.), *Holistic nursing: a handbook for practice* (p. 209–228). Sudbury, MA: Jones and Bartlett Publishers.

Maytum, J. C., Heiman, M. B., & Garwick, A. W. (2004). Compassion fatigue and burnout in nurses who work with children with chronic conditions and their families. *Pediatric Health Care*, 18(4), 171–179.

Meadors, P., Lamson, A., Swanson, M., White, M., & Sira, N. (2009). Secondary traumatization in pediatric healthcare providers: Compassion fatigue, burnout, and secondary traumatic stress. *OMEGA—Journal of Death and Dying*, 60(2), 103–128.

Moore, A., & Malinowski, P. (2009). Meditation, mindfulness and cognitive flexibility. *Consciousness and Cognition*, 18, 176–186. doi:10.1016/j.concog.2008.12.008

Mostofsky, E., Maclure, M., Sherwood, J. B., Tofler, G. H., Muller, J. E., & Mittleman, M. A. (2012). Risk of acute myocardial infarction after the death of a significant person on one's life: The determinants of myocardial infarction onset study. *Circulation*, 125(3), 491–496. doi: 10.1161/CIRCULATIONAHA.111.061770. Epub 2012 Jan 9.

National Institutes of Health (2013). *Antioxidants*. Bethesda, MD: Author. Retrieved from: http://www.nlm.nih.gov/medlineplus/antioxidants.html

Nevins, N. (2013). *Benefits of yoga*. Retrieved from http://www.osteopathic.org/osteopathic-health/about-your-health/health-conditions-library/general-health/Pages/yoga.aspx.

Ortner, C. N. M., Kilner, S. J., & Zelazo, P. D. (2007). Mindfulness meditation and reduced emotional interference on a cognitive task. *Motivation and Emotion*, 31, 271–283. doi: 10.1007/s11031-007-9076-7.

Park, Y., Subar, A. F., Hollenbeck, A., & Schatzkin, A. (2011). Dietary fiber intake and mortality in the NIH-AARP diet and health study. *Archives of Internal Medicine*, 171(12), 1061–1068.

Pate, R. R., Pratt, M., Blair, S. N., Haskell, W. L., Macera, C. A., Bouchard, C, ... King, A. C. (1995). Physical activity and public health. A recommendation from the Centers for Disease Control and Prevention and the American College of Sports Medicine. *Journal of the American Medical Association*, 273, 402–407.

Richardson, C. (2009). *The art of extreme self-care*. Carlsbad, CA: Hay House.

Rogers, A. E. (2008). The effects of fatigue and sleepiness on nurse performance and patient safety. In R. G. Hughes (Ed.), *Patient safety and quality: An evidence-based handbook for nurses.* (Chapter 40). Rockville, MD: Agency for Healthcare Research and Quality.

Sabo, B. M. (2006). Compassion fatigue and nursing work: Can we accurately capture the consequences of caring work? *International Journal of Nursing Practice*, 12, 136–142.

Schaub, R., & Schaub, B. (2013). *Transpersonal development: Cultivating the human resources of peace, wisdom, purpose and oneness*. Huntington, NY: Florence Press.

Seligman, M. E. P. (2002). *Authentic happiness: Using the new positive psychology to realize your potential for lasting fulfillment*. New York: Free Press.

Showalter, S. E. (2010). Compassion fatigue: What is it? Why does it matter? Recognizing the symptoms, acknowledging the impact, developing the tools to prevent compassion fatigue and strengthen the professional already suffering from the effects. *American Journal of Hospice and Palliative Medicine*, 27(4), 239–242.

Siegel, D. J. (2007). Mindfulness training and neural integration: Differentiation of distinct streams of awareness and the cultivation of well-being. *Social Cognitive and Affective Neuroscience*, 2, 259–263. doi:10.1093/scan/nsm034

Singh, M., Drake, C. L., Roehrs, T., Hudgel, D. W., & Roth, T. (2005). The association between obesity and short sleep duration: a population-based study. *Journal of Clinical Sleep Medicine: Official publication of the American Academy of Sleep Medicine*, 1(4), 357–363.

Smith, D. (2012). *Monkey mind: A memoir of anxiety*. New York: Simon & Schuster.

Spiegel, K., Leproult, R., & Van Cauter, E. (1999). Impact of sleep debt on metabolic and endocrine functions. *Lancet, 354*(9188), 1435–1439.

Tai Chi Research (2014). Retrieved from http://www.taichiresearch.com/

Thomas, R. B., & Wilson, J. P. (2004). Issues and controversies in the understanding of compassion fatigue, vicarious traumatization and secondary traumatic stress disorder. *International Journal of Emergency Mental Health*, 6(2), 81–92.

Thompson, P. D., Buchner, D., Piña, I., Balady, G., Williams, M., Marcus, B., ... Wenger, N. (2003). Exercise and physical activity in the prevention and treatment of atherosclerotic cardiovascular disease. *Circulation,* 107, 3109-3116. doi:10.1161/01. CIR.0000075572.40158.77

Trichopoulou, A., Bamia, C., Lagiou, P., & Trichopoulos, D. (2010). Conformity to traditional Mediterranean diet and breast cancer risk in the Greek EPIC (European Prospective Investigation into Cancer and Nutrition) cohort. *American Journal of Clinical Nutrition,* 92(3), 620–625. doi:10.3945/ajcn.2010.29619

Tsivgoulis, G., Judd, S., Letter, A., Alexandrov, A., Howard, G., Nahab, F., ... Wadley, V. (2013). Adherence to a Mediterranean diet and risk of incident cognitive impairment. *Neurology,* 80(18), 1684–1692. doi: 10.1212/WNL.0b013e3182904f69

United States Department of Agriculture. (2010). *Report of the dietary guidelines advisory committee on the dietary guidelines for Americans, 2010*. Washington, DC: U. S. Department of Agriculture. Retrieved from http://www.cnpp.usda.gov/ dgas2010-dgacreport.htm

United States Department of Health and Human Services. (2008). *Physical activity guidelines for Americans.* Washington, DC: U.S. Department of Health and Human Services. Retrieved from http://www.health.gov/paguidelines/guidelines/

Walsh, R., & Shapiro, S. L. (2006). The meeting of meditative disciplines and western psychology: A mutually enriching dialogue. *American Psychologist,* 61, 227–239. doi:10.1037/0003-066X.61.3.227

Wang, C., Bannuru, R., Ramel, J., Kupelnick, B., Scott, T., & Schmid, C. H. (2010). Tai Chi on psychological well-being: Systematic review and meta-analysis. *BMC Complementary and Alternative Medicine,* 10(23). doi:10.1186/1472-6882-10-23. Retrieved from http://www.ncbi.nlm.nih.gov/pmc/articles/PMC2893078/

Wellman, N. S., Kamp, B., Kirk-Sanchez, N. J., & Johnson, P. M. (2007). Eat better & move more: a community-based program designed to improve diets and increase physical activity among older Americans. *American Journal of Public Health,* 97(4), 710–717. Epub 2007 Feb 28.

Wieder, S. (2011). *Tips for working with an accountability buddy*. British Columbia: Youngblood Coaching. Retrieved from http://www.youngbloodcoaching.com/ accountability-buddy.html

Yang, K. (2007). A review of yoga programs for four leading risk factors of chronic diseases. *Evidenced Based Complementary and Alternative Medicine,* 4(4), 487–491. doi:10.1093/ecam/nem154

Yoder, E. A. (2010). Compassion fatigue in nurses. *Applied Nursing Research,* 23(4), 191–197.

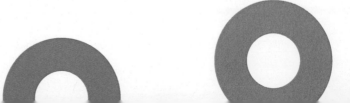

Your self-care notes: Pathways and progress

_____

_____

_____

_____

Physical Self-care

_____

_____

_____

_____

_____

Mental Self-care

_____

_____

_____

_____

_____

Emotional Self-care

_____

_____

_____

_____

_____

Spiritual Self-care

_____

_____

_____

_____

_____

Relationship Self-care

_____

_____

_____

_____

_____

Choice Self-care

_____

_____

_____

_____

_____

Self-care progress

_____

_____

_____

_____

_____